DR Garth Pettit

STOP
THE ROT

Stop Telling Children "Brush Your Teeth"

Morgan James Publishing • New York

Dr. Garth Pettit

STOP
THE ROT

Library of Congress Control Number: 1600375421
ISBN: 978-1-60037-542-2   (Paperback)

Published by:
Morgan James Publishing, LLC
1225 Franklin Avenue Suite 325
Garden City, NY 11530-1693

Toll Free 800-485-4943
www.MorganJamesPublishing.com

Cover & Interior Design by:
3 Dog Design
www.3dogdesign.net

General Editor:
Heather Campbell

Illustrations By:
Richard Coburn - Art Media Productions
rwcoburn@aapt.net.au

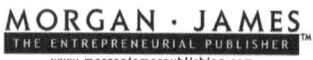

MORGAN · JAMES™
THE ENTREPRENEURIAL PUBLISHER
www.morganjamespublishing.com

Habitat
for Humanity®
Peninsula
Building Partner

contents

preface

"They always say time changes things, but you actually have to change them yourself"

Andy Warhol (1928 – 1987), The Philosophy of Andy Warhol

This book presents reasons and needs for making changes to a hygiene instruction that has its origins in the fifteenth century, specifically, the reasons and needs for changing the tooth-cleaning instruction to "Brush Your Teeth."

Brush Your Teeth has remained intact, word for word, for over five hundred years. It may well have existed side by side with additional and since-forgotten hygiene instructions, but there was never a change in the name of the instruction itself.

Compared with five hundred years ago, we now live in a world with vastly improved knowledge of hygiene, including oral hygiene. Brush Your Teeth is a hygiene instruction, but not in the full sense of our current understanding of hygiene. Brush Your Teeth is only a part of a total mouth, oral hygiene instruction. There are many more surfaces in the mouth, besides tooth surfaces, that must be considered in relation to oral hygiene and an oral hygiene instruction.

Children in this twenty-first century are instructed to Brush Your Teeth by their parents on an average of twice each day. At other times, teachers at school instruct children to Brush Your Teeth, visiting grandparents instruct children to Brush Your Teeth, dentists instruct children to Brush Your Teeth, dental therapists instruct children to Brush Your Teeth, and dental hygienists reinforce the instruction to Brush Your Teeth. Many oral health promotions promote the instruction to Brush Your Teeth. To achieve and maintain oral health, children are instructed to Brush Your Teeth over and over again.

From the early age of four through their midteens, children are told to Brush Your Teeth. By the time a four–year-old child becomes a sixteen-year-old teenager, the child may well have been told to Brush Your Teeth twice each day for seven days each week for fifty-two weeks each year for thirteen years. Instructing a child to Brush Your Teeth 9,464 times is a lot of repetition. It actually amounts to *brainwashing*! What does that child do for the rest of his or her life? Brush Your Teeth, of course! Often, despite whatever else he or she may have been told, Brush Your Teeth alone dominates his or her memory.

The goal of Brush Your Teeth is to avert all easily preventable oral diseases such as tooth decay, gum diseases, bad breath, and stained teeth, thereby preventing the need for dental treatments. But the truth is, thousands of people around the world who have been instructed to Brush Your Teeth visit dentists every day, keeping dentists busy with the treatment of easily preventable oral diseases. The need for most treatments is evidence that Brush Your Teeth is *not* preventing oral diseases. Some treatments may be accounted for by patients' nonconformity to Brush Your Teeth. However, there is evidence that even patient conformity does not always prevent the need for dental treatment.

Ask yourself these questions after reading this book:

- Can the instruction to Brush Your Teeth contribute to easily preventable oral diseases?

- Has Brush Your Teeth prevented your need for dental treatments throughout life?

- Has Brush Your Teeth prevented your family's need for dental treatments throughout life?

- Has Brush Your Teeth prevented your friends' need for dental treatments throughout life?

- Has Brush Your Teeth led to a lifetime of oral health for anyone you know?

- Do you think Brush Your Teeth will give today's children their best chance to enjoy the benefits of oral health without the need for dental treatment and only a need for regular check-ups?

This book gives you the details of my strongly recommended, twenty-first century, oral hygiene instruction, an alternative to the fifteenth century Brush Your Teeth. I believe it to be the first-ever serious contender.

Only you can make the suggested changes to banish the tooth-cleaning instruction to Brush Your Teeth and to adopt in its place the more appropriate, twenty-first century, oral hygiene instruction that I suggest in this book.

about the author

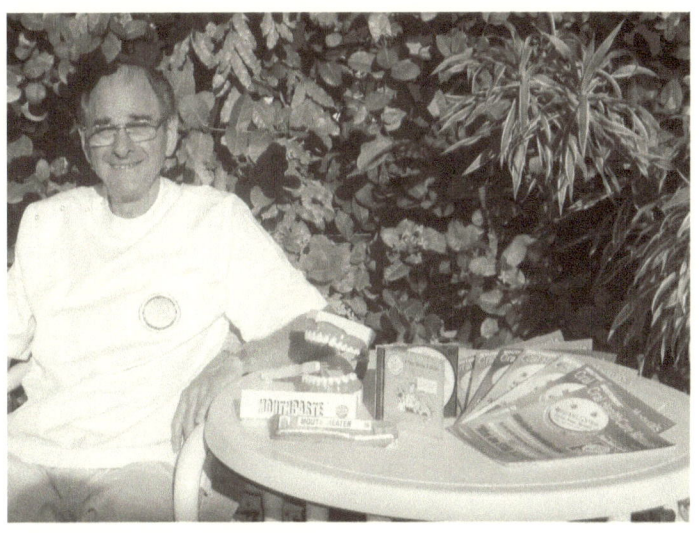

My MouthWise™ Oral HealthCare Advice and
MouthWise Oral Hygiene Instruction for Children
To Prevent Oral Diseases is

"Treat Your Whole Mouth"

introduction

Hello Readers,

Everyday life is filled with examples of following instructions that have long since become habits. Habitually following an instruction creates the tendency to do it automatically and to do it without thinking, even without the need for thinking. Brush Your Teeth is a classic example of such an instruction. Twice in recent months, in emails to me from eminent Internet marketers, the statement to Brush Your Teeth has been used to imply it is a no-brainer, requiring no thinking. I beg to differ.

My cover page statements are profound and alarming, aren't they?

- Stop "the Rot"

- Stop telling children to Brush Your Teeth

- Brush Your Teeth is a cause of oral disease

The Rot above is my reference to the unacceptably high and seemingly endless incidences of oral disease found in people of all ages over a very long period of time. In fact, the Rot has been occurring from generation to generation for five hundred years. Throughout this span of time, documentation of dental treatments recorded by dentists consistently included proof of the Rot. And there is little evidence early in the twenty-first century of the Rot abating.[1]

In the following pages, I hope to convince you that all three statements are urgently in need of your attention and, especially in the best interests of children, require your action.

After graduating in November 1953 from the University of Adelaide, I was in general dental practice until retiring in November 1992. Throughout that entire period, my advice to all patients was Brush Your Teeth but with the added instruction "and your gums around your teeth." Because of the far-from-desirable results it returned, I, like most dentists, blamed continuing oral disease on noncompliant patients. I mutely criticized the value of most oral health, handout pamphlets, considering them as totally inadequate in preventing oral diseases. It was many years later before my thoughts focused on preventing oral disease in children.

In 1996, my youngest grandchild succumbed to tooth decay from sucking on a bottle of milk at night. Horrified, blaming myself for my grandchild's suffering, I decided to return to work to create and publish oral healthcare education resources for people of all age groups.

But even then, my resources were to be based on the instruction to Brush Your Teeth and a character I had named "Toothee Brush." At that point in time, I had no reasons to do otherwise. I thought, because of my grand-child's decayed tooth, that the first resource I published would be for young children.

In January 1997, I was accepted for a position as a district dental officer in a government dental clinic where I worked with primary school–aged children and their teachers, schools, and parents.

The first resources for young children were not ready for publishing until early 2002. The manuscripts were turned down by several book publishers in Australia (each time I was told there was "no market for them"!), which eventually resulted in my decision to self-publish.

1. The University of Adelaide, "Early tooth decay in children increasing," *The University of Adelaide*, www.adelaide.edu.au/news/news6983.html.

CHAPTER 1

Traditional Oral Hygiene Advice

Traditional oral hygiene advice has been and still is, "Brush Your Teeth." But not in the future if my advice is taken.

Let me quote from an article I read recently on the internet:

On January 22nd 2003, the results of a new survey conducted by the Lemelson – MIT Invention Index at the Massachusetts Institute of Technology, which asked which of 5 inventions Americans could not live without, were released.

The toothbrush emerged the undisputed champion beating the car, the personal computer, the cell phone and the microwave...in that order...as the most prized innovation.[1, 2]

However, I firmly believe that very few children, or adults for that matter, have ever received advice on and instructions on how to use the toothbrush in the most effective manner, which would achieve a state of oral hygiene that would in turn, most predictably, prevent simple oral diseases such as tooth decay, gum diseases, bad breath, and stained teeth.[2]

The inability of children to use a toothbrush in the most effective manner to prevent oral disease has been a cause, is still a cause, and will continue to be a cause, of oral disease in children.

Hygiene, according to the *Oxford Popular Dictionary*, is "cleanliness as a means of preventing disease."

Oral hygiene advice is how-to information given to a person to help that person to reach and maintain a state of oral hygiene in his or her mouth that will be sufficiently effective in the prevention of common oral diseases such as tooth decay, gum disease, bad breath, and stained teeth, all of which are described by the dental profession as easily preventable oral diseases.

In the fifteenth century, or possibly before, there emerged the instruction to Brush Your Teeth. It was a very basic hygiene instruction, a tooth-only and cleaning-only instruction. The evidence of this advice dates back to June 26, 1498, in the form of an invention by a Chinese emperor of the first-ever "toothbrush made with bristles." He set the bristles at right angles to a bone or bamboo handle. The chewing-sticks used previously had frayed ends from chewing the end of a twig.[3-7]

Since the fifteenth century, children have continued to be instructed by various combinations of advisors, parents, teachers, dentists, toothbrush manufacturers and dentifrice manufacturers, and others in the oral healthcare industry to Brush Your Teeth. The medium used in the fifteenth century, in conjunction with the toothbrush, to achieve cleaning was salt, sand, or charcoal. Toothpastes had not then been invented. Dr Julien Botot, a Frenchman, is credited with inventing the first toothpaste for Louis XV of France in 1755, the same year he also invented the first mouthwash for the king.[8]

Early in the twentieth century, advice was given to also use the toothbrush to clean the gums adjacent to the teeth. This gum is called gingiva (singular) or gingivae (plural). Gingivitis is inflammation of the gingival or gingivae. Then advice to use a toothbrush to clean the tongue as well came later in the twentieth century.

Modern manufacturers of toothpaste claimed the ingredients in their products would clean teeth, gums, and the tongue and offer protection to prevent and repair tooth decay, prevent gum diseases and bad breath, kill bacteria, and prevent plaque and scale.

But, just as for the humble toothbrush, the how-to-use instructions for toothpastes were either nonexistent or lamentably poor. Instructions were absent on packaging; given instead by word of mouth from dentists, parents, and teachers and easily forgotten or misinterpreted. Parents had very little idea themselves about how to effectively use a toothbrush and toothpaste, so how could they give their children the advice needed to prevent oral diseases?

Then new and improved mouthwash products appeared on the market, some of which were given a seal of approval and recommended by dental associations. The suggested use for these products was to follow brushing your teeth with toothpaste with rinsing your mouth with mouthwash to prevent oral diseases. But mouthwashes offered the same benefits as toothpaste. So I asked myself, what was wrong with the toothpastes that they needed a supplement? Why was toothpaste alone not achieving the prevention of oral diseases that was claimed and intended? My answer was simple—because an ideal instruction for using a toothbrush and toothpaste had never been offered.

Brush Your Teeth has traditionally been followed by the often unspoken advice to "then rinse your mouth" (with water). Late in the twentieth century, in an attempt to achieve oral hygiene and to stem the incidence of tooth decay, not rinsing with water after brushing the teeth was advised by some school dental services. The intent was to leave the toothpaste ingredients in the mouth for maximum benefit. But, logically, you have to rinse to get rid of the dirt from the mouth, so leaving the mouth dirty while leaving toothpaste in the mouth amounted to, in my opinion, poor oral hygiene advice. However, the vast majority of people continued to just brush and rinse, probably because that advice never reached them.

There exists abundant, well-documented evidence eight years into the twenty-first century that all easily preventable oral diseases continue to be of great concern in all age groups, not just in children.[9] Despite fluoridation measures, fissure sealants, countless oral health promotions, public education programs, and increasing numbers of dental graduates, there are not enough dentists to cope with the high demands for treatment. Dentists every day, all over the world, are kept busy with the treatment of oral diseases caused by the instruction to Brush Your Teeth.

Maybe it is time to question the value of the instruction and the advice that has been given. After all, Brush Your Teeth was and still is a fifteenth-century instruction!

Doing research for the books I was writing for children made me do just that: I questioned the value of the instruction to Brush Your Teeth.

In a following chapter, "Two Special Teachers in East Arnhem," I describe how I discovered that Brush Your Teeth was of dubious value in preventing oral diseases such as tooth decay, gum diseases, bad breath, and stained teeth.

1. Jeordan Legon, "Toothbrush trounces car as top invention," *CNN.com,* www.cnn.com/2003/TECH/ptech/01/22/toothbrush.king.
2. The Mobi Blog.com, "101 Gadgets That Changed the World," *The Mobi Blog.com,* www.themobiblog.com/2007/11/101-gadgets-that-changed-world.html.
3. www.todayinsci.com/6/6_26.htm.
4. www.a0kteacherstuff.com/Jun_calendar.htm.
5. www.26june.info.
6. www.dentalcarefind.com/dentalcare/toothbrushes.html.
7. www.danb.org/PDFs/CPSummer03.pdf.
8. www.letrainblue.com/botottoothpaste.aspx.
9. www.arcpoh.adelaide.edu.au/publications/report/research/pdf_files/rr6_nursinghomes.pdf.

CHAPTER 2

Two Special Teachers in East Arnhem

Here is a quote from a page on one of my websites. Oral Health Help Site, http://www.oralhealthhelpsite.com.

Hello, I am the author, Garth Pettit, or better known to children as GarGar The Dentist. It is appropriate that this story about two very special teachers who taught at a remote Australian Aboriginal Community School in Numbulwar, East Arnhem Land, be given a special page on this website to acknowledge their very special, un-witting contribution to exposing the problems associated with the oral hygiene instruction, "Brush Your Teeth."

I chose to call these two teachers "special teachers" because they, although inadvertently, were responsible for my creation of a new and more appropriate oral hygiene instruction than Brush Your Teeth.

I visited many East Arnhem Land schools regularly over a period of more than five years (1997–2002). Every year, in each East Arnhem Land school, children were subjected to a screening for decayed, missing, and filled teeth. The screenings at the beginning of the year revealed massive oral disease problems in the vast majority of children in these schools. The remainder of the year was spent attempting to treat as much oral disease as possible. But the Numbulwar school screenings exhibited a different oral disease pattern from all the other schools.

The Numbulwar school children in two classrooms of six- to eight-year-old children did not have rotten teeth, bleeding gums, or bad breath as was found in all the other classrooms. After witnessing this phenomenon repeated over a two-to-three-year period, I approached the two teachers, told them what I had witnessed, and asked them if they could explain what they did differently from other classrooms.

The two teachers responsible for these children had proudly taken it upon themselves to create a breakfast regime. This consisted of giving their students a healthy breakfast before the first lesson started. They certainly would not have had that at home before leaving for school because rarely does an Australian Aboriginal child have a breakfast and even more rarely a healthy one. After breakfast, they instructed the children to Brush Your Teeth at one of the outside verandah water troughs.

I was not satisfied with this explanation, so I asked for more details and discovered that they instructed the children to "Brush your teeth and rinse and rinse and rinse your brush under the tap." This was now beginning to make sense to me. In my early years in dentistry, I treated many Aboriginal patients and recalled that Aboriginal people take instructions literally. I then deduced correctly what was making their mouths so different.

The Aboriginal language is very precise. The children interpreted their teachers' instructions literally. They were *brushing their teeth* and then they were *rinsing and rinsing and rinsing their brush under the tap*. The teachers meant for the children to *brush your teeth and rinse your mouth* and then *rinse and rinse your brush under the tap*.

By not rinsing their mouths, they were leaving behind a coating of toothpaste on their teeth, gums and tongue.

The result was quite remarkable. Their incidence of arrested decay (old decay that has become inactive) rose dramatically. Their incidence of new dental decay fell to virtually zero. Their gums were healthier. Their tongues were healthier, and their breath was fresher. Why? Fortunately, my knowledge and experience with Aboriginal people allowed me to answer this.

By not rinsing their mouths, they were leaving toothpaste in their mouths. The ingredients in the toothpaste were causing this dramatic, beneficial effect on their teeth and on their gums and on their tongues. Their whole mouths were healthier. Children in classes below them, with no breakfast regime, exhibited the usual high rates of decay. Children in classes above them, with no breakfast regime, exhibited dramatically increased rates of decay.

However, I still held the opinion that, by not rinsing with water, dirt from both the brushed surfaces and the not-brushed surfaces was being left in the mouth, and that was definitely not desirable for oral hygiene. Eventually, it dawned upon me that I had to rewrite the oral hygiene instruction to Brush Your Teeth. It was misleading and *outdated*! I pondered for weeks about creating the new and superior oral hygiene instruction to "Treat Your Mouth."

Future generations of children who learn to treat their mouths from an early age and who will then benefit from a lifetime of oral health will have much to thank for those two special teachers' unwitting, but exceedingly valuable, contribution to the prevention of oral diseases, tooth decay, gum diseases, bad breath, and stained teeth.

CHAPTER 3

21st Century MouthWise Oral Hygiene Advice

The primary objective of oral hygiene advice is to help a person to attain and to maintain a state of oral health by giving advice based on the best knowledge available at the time. The Chinese emperor who invented the first ever toothbrush made with bristles used every bit of scientific knowledge available to him at that time when creating that first bristle made toothbrush.

That oral health is an essential part of general health, and in some facets of general health a very critical factor, is well recorded. Knowledge in the twenty-first century contributes to oral health just as knowledge contributed to oral health in the fifteenth century. It would be ludicrous to doubt that twenty-first-century knowledge of oral hygiene has not progressed beyond the fifteenth century. So why still Brush Your Teeth? Why no change?

In 1996, I had been retired from dentistry for four years but decided, when my youngest grandchild developed tooth decay, to return to work to write a series of oral healthcare education resources. This is when I made the astonishing discovery that the instruction to Brush Your Teeth was of questionable value. I had to devise a new and better oral hygiene instruction. I decided to rewrite the resources that I had based on Brush Your Teeth and my character "Toothee Brush" but not yet published. I decided to do a SWOT test (strength, weakness, opportunity, threat) on Brush Your Teeth.

For the first time ever, I began to think deeply about the following questions:

- What are the objectives of an ideal oral hygiene instruction?

- What oral hygiene instruction will best achieve these objectives?

- What is the best advice I can give to my patients to execute the instruction and achieve these objectives?

I developed a set of new oral hygiene instructions, assembled these instructions into a sequence, and chose the name "Treat Your Mouth" for the new advice. I then rewrote the oral healthcare education resources.

I chose the trademark "MouthWise" for the resources. The first resource, *The MouthWise Oral HealthCare Manual 2*, together with a CD titled *4 Your Smile 2 Shine*, were self-published in mid-2002. They are now marketed as *The Mouth-Wise Oral Health Kit*, educational resources for children five years to eleven years, their parents, and their teachers.

I have more recently changed the instruction from Treat Your Mouth to "Treat Your Whole Mouth" to clearly convey the message that, when eating or drinking, every surface of every structure within the mouth gets dirty and must be cleaned. After this cleaning, the surfaces then need to be protected.

Treat Your Whole Mouth is a two-step oral hygiene instruction. It is an ideal oral hygiene instruction because the first step gets rid of dirt from the whole mouth by cleaning every surface with bristles and the detergent ingredient in the paste. Then, in the second step, the bristles are used to paint the active ingredients in the paste onto vulnerable surfaces to prevent oral diseases.

The surfaces to be cleaned in the first step of Treat Your Whole Mouth include the following:

- Teeth surfaces

- Gum surfaces

- Tongue surfaces

- Roof of the mouth

- Floor of the mouth under the tongue

- The inside surfaces of the cheeks

- The inside surfaces of the lips

But just cleaning these surfaces does not protect them from oral diseases. These surfaces must also be protected, particularly the surfaces of the teeth, gums, and tongue. This is the second required step to Treat Your Whole Mouth—protecting surfaces from oral diseases.

These are the surfaces that are protected by the second step:

- Teeth

- Gums

- Tongue

CHAPTER 4

Treat Your Whole Mouth

The intention of an oral hygiene instruction is to help prevent oral diseases. Preventing oral diseases is not a passive process.

In the fifteenth century, processed foods played little part in a daily diet, but sugar was beginning to have its detrimental effects on teeth, especially on the very noticeable, top front teeth. Hence, the instruction, Brush Your Teeth, to clean teeth.

In the twenty-first century, the prevention of oral diseases has become an active vigilance because of the proliferation of processed foods, especially that of sugar-laden processed foods and drinks and the detrimental effects they have on the teeth, gums, and tongues. The oral hygiene

15

instruction to Treat Your Whole Mouth addresses all the issues that threaten oral health in the twenty-first century.

Unlike Brush Your Teeth, Treat Your Whole Mouth is

- A twenty-first century oral hygiene instruction, not a fifteenth century instruction.

- An instruction that is a totally oral, oral hygiene instruction, that includes all surfaces in the mouth, as opposed to an instruction that refers to teeth only.

- An instruction that sets out to achieve total hygiene in the whole mouth as a means of preventing disease as opposed to just cleanliness of tooth surfaces only.

- A two-step instruction. The first step is advice to treat the mouth using the bristles of the mouthtreater (my preferred name for a toothbrush) and the detergent ingredient in the mouthpaste (my preferred name for toothpaste) to clean the whole mouth. The second step is advice to treat the mouth using the bristles of the mouthtreater and the active ingredients in the mouthpaste to treat the whole mouth again. This ensures two highly desirable conditions: optimum oral hygiene and optimum protection from oral diseases. This two-step instruction is far superior to just cleaning one surface, the teeth, and then rinsing and leaving the whole mouth vulnerable to oral disease.

CHAPTER 5

MouthTreater and MouthPaste

Nomenclature, according to the dictionary, is a "system of names, such as in science."

An instruction, any instruction, should precisely and clearly indicate the desired objective, the method by which that desired objective can be achieved, and the tools and materials that will be used to achieve it.

An oral hygiene instruction in the twenty-first century that has the objective of preventing oral diseases with the instruction to Treat Your Whole Mouth cannot logically include nomenclature such as "with a toothbrush" and "with toothpaste": these phrases are relics from the fifteenth century. Treat Your Whole Mouth requires new nomenclature.

Advising a child to Treat Your Whole Mouth with a toothbrush and toothpaste is illogical. These names from the past would not help a child to think clearly about the new instruction. It makes more sense to rename the brush and the paste. Treat Your Whole Mouth with a *mouthtreater* and *mouthpaste*. I believe these new words will help children to think more clearly about what they are trying to accomplish and also help them to achieve a better result. Treat Your Whole Mouth with a mouthtreater and mouthpaste to prevent oral diseases.

My advice that follows is very simple, and it is nothing more than how best to use bristles and paste ingredients inside your mouth to achieve your objectives—prevent easily preventable oral diseases such as tooth decay, gum diseases, bad breath, and stained teeth.

Incidentally, but very importantly, my advice will also prevent the need for many expensive visits to dentists, but you will still need the regular inexpensive visits for routine examinations.

The next chapter begins the detailed instructions for Treat Your Whole Mouth with a mouthtreater and mouthpaste to clean every surface in your mouth that gets dirty every time you eat and or drink and to protect every surface that is vulnerable to common oral diseases.

CHAPTER 6

Treat Upper Jaw to Clean Surfaces

Step 1
Your First Treat Cleaning The Upper Jaw

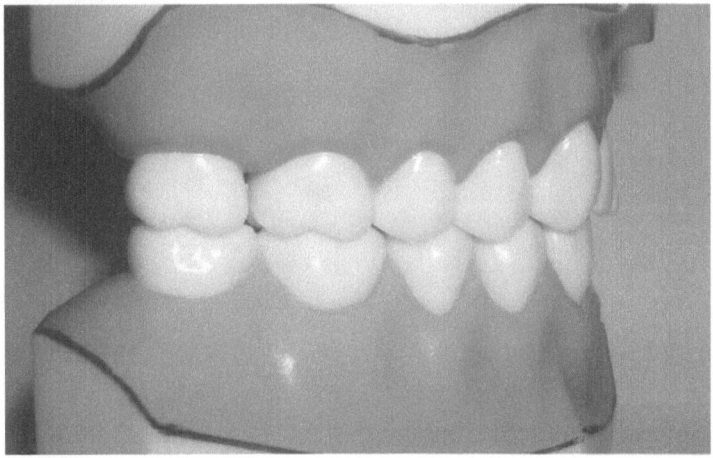

Fig. 6.1. Outside surfaces of posterior teeth and gums and upper and lower jaws. Photo by Richard Coburn

If you open wide, your cheek muscles will be taut and you will only be able to get back as far as your first molar teeth. To get to the very back teeth, top and bottom and both sides close your mouth slightly, let the muscles of your cheeks and lips relax. Then you can get the bristles and paste to the very back teeth and gums easily.

Step 2

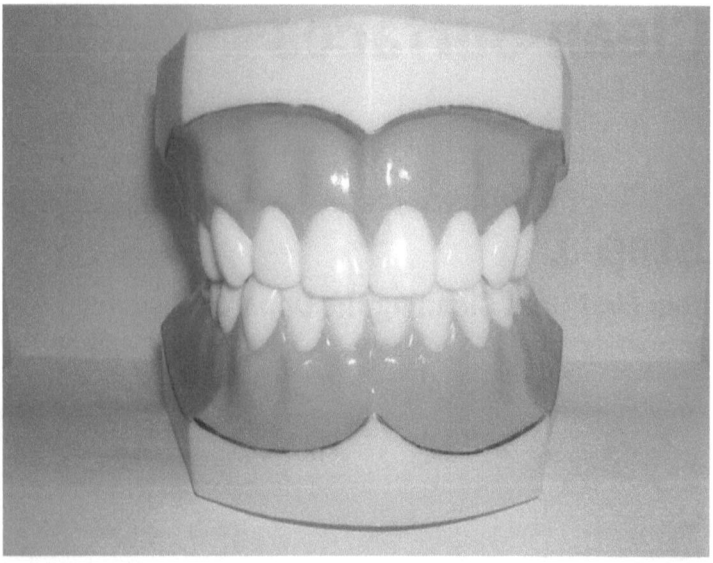

Fig. 6.2. Outside teeth and gum surfaces of front teeth
Photo by Richard Coburn

Hold the mouthtreater horizontally and move the bristles up and down vertically across the entire tooth surfaces and the entire gum surfaces up as far as the cheek or in the front up as far as the lip.

Continue all the way around from last molar tooth on one side across the front teeth and until you reach the last molar tooth on the other side.

Next, open wide, holding the mouthtreater horizontally with handle forward. Pass the bristles backwards and forwards across the chewing surfaces of your back teeth, both sides. Then move the bristles from side to side across the back surface of the last tooth and gum behind it on each side.

Step 3

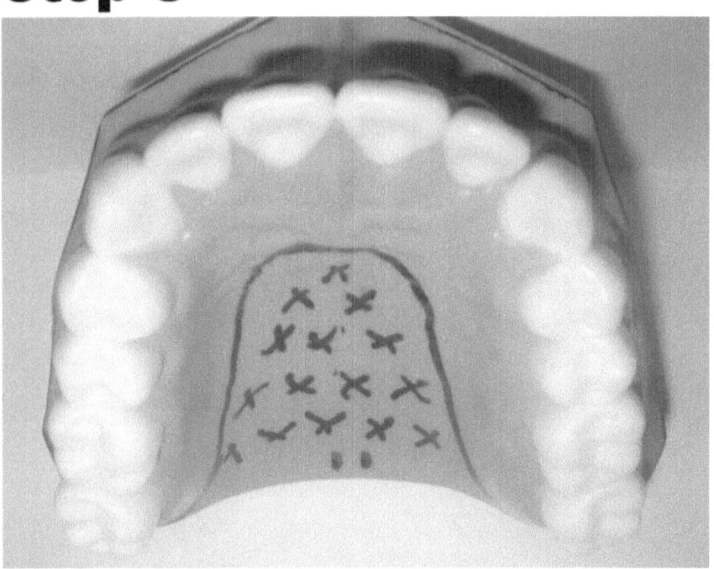

Fig. 6.3. Upper jaw: Chewing and inside surfaces of the teeth, gums, and roof of the mouth Photo by Richard Coburn

Next are the inside surfaces of your top teeth and gums. Hold the mouthtreater vertically, handle down. Move the bristles across the surfaces of the teeth and across the gum to where the gum and the roof surfaces join. Continue all the way round from one side to the other.

Then move the bristles from side to side across the roof of your mouth.

CHAPTER **7**

Treat Lower Jaw to Clean Surfaces

Step 4
Next, Your First Treat Cleaning The Lower Jaw

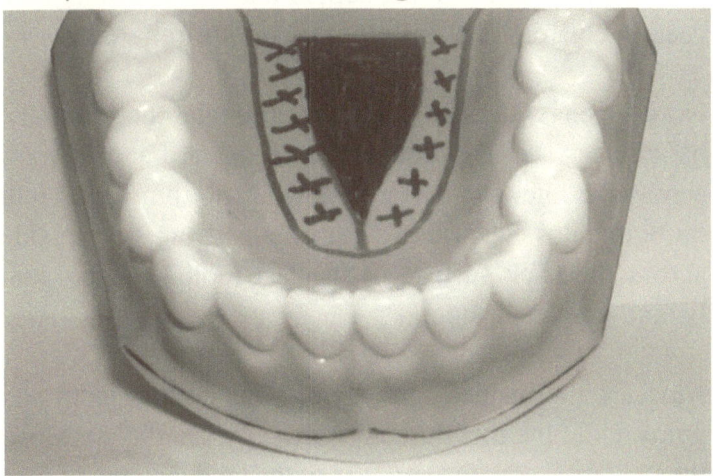

Fig. 7.1. Lower jaw: Outside and inside surfaces of teeth and gums, chewing surfaces, the floor of the mouth, and each side under the tongue. Photo by Richard Coburn

Next, you will treat the outside surfaces of your bottom teeth and gums. Remember to close your mouth a little to relax your cheek and lip muscles to enable the bristles to reach across the entire surfaces of the very back teeth and gum down to where the gum joins the cheeks or the lip.

Hold the mouthtreater horizontally, handle forward, and move the bristles up and down vertically across the entire tooth surfaces and the entire gum surfaces, down as far as the cheek. Continue all the way around from the last molar tooth on one side, across the front teeth, down to the lip, and to the last molar tooth on the other side.

Note particularly that you must relax your lip muscles to enable the bristles to reach down to the bottom of your gums; otherwise, as most people do, you will only succeed in cleaning the tips of your bottom front teeth.

Now, open wide. Hold the mouthtreater horizontally, handle forward. Pass the bristles backward and forward across the chewing surfaces of your bottom back teeth on both sides. Then move the bristles from side to side across the back surface of the last tooth and the gum behind it on each side.

Next are the insides surfaces of your bottom teeth and gums. Hold the mouthtreater vertically, handle up. Move the bristles across the surfaces of the teeth and well down across the gum to the floor of the mouth, all the way round from one side to the other. Pay particular attention to the inside of the bottom front teeth surfaces because this is a very common place for plaque to be left behind and then for scale to form.

Then treat under the tongue and across the floor of your mouth on each side by holding the mouthtreater horizontally, handle forward, and passing the bristles from front to back across the floor.

CHAPTER **8**

Treat Tongue, Cheeks & Lips to Clean Surfaces

Step 5
End Your First Treat Cleaning Tongue, Cheeks & Lips

Next, poke out your tongue and, starting at the tip, pass the bristles from side to side across the tongue. Repeat this for as far back as you can tolerate. Then clean the tongue from front to back, again as far back as you can tolerate.

Next, clean the inside surfaces of the left cheek. Hold the handle horizontally with the bristles facing toward the left cheek. Close your lips. Now rotate the handle to move the bristles across the inside left cheek surface.

Next, clean the inside surfaces of the right cheek. Hold the handle horizontally with the bristles facing toward the right cheek. Close your lips and rotate the handle to move the bristles across the inside right cheek surface.

Next, clean the inside top lip surface. Hold the handle vertically, bristles up and handle down, with the bristles facing the inside top lip surface. Sweep the bristles from left to right across the inside lip surface two or three times.

Finally, clean the inside bottom lip surface. Hold handle vertically, bristles down and handle up, with the bristles facing the inside bottom lip surface. Sweep the bristles from left to right across the inside lip surface two or three times.

CHAPTER 9

Complete First Treat to Leave Mouth Clean

Step 6

Every surface within your mouth has now been brushed with the bristles and detergent in the paste to clean every surface.

The detergent agent in the mouthpaste has trapped all the dirty substances that were left in the mouth after eating and drinking. These substances are now suspended in the liquid within the mouth and need to be expelled.

Thorough rinsing with water and spitting the water out, over and over again, is the most efficient way to achieve this.

Besides filling the mouth with water from a glass or cupped hand, it is also helpful to "load" the bristles with water. Place the water-laden bristles inside the mouth with the bristles facing toward the outside surfaces of the left back teeth and then close your lips and cheeks. Next, slightly open the left cheek and suck air into the mouth. This action will draw water from the water-laden bristles between the upper and lower teeth to flush out the dirt between the teeth. Repeat this process for the outside surfaces of the right back teeth as well.

Now, repeat this for the outside surfaces of the front teeth. Of course, this time keep your cheeks closed and open only the lips slightly.

Every surface in the whole mouth is now clean. Pristine clean! But they are not protected. Remember, the mouthpaste has gone with the dirt!

At this point, let me remind you that the objective is to prevent oral diseases by protecting the vulnerable surfaces in your mouth. So far, you have only made use of the paste's detergent ingredient. You now need to use the other important ingredients in the paste to provide the protection.

Treat Your Whole Mouth simply uses bristles and paste ingredients with greatly increased efficiency compared to the Brush Your Teeth regime.

CHAPTER **10**

Treat Top Teeth, Gums to Prevent Diseases

Step 1
Your Second Treat Paint On The Mouthpaste Ingredients

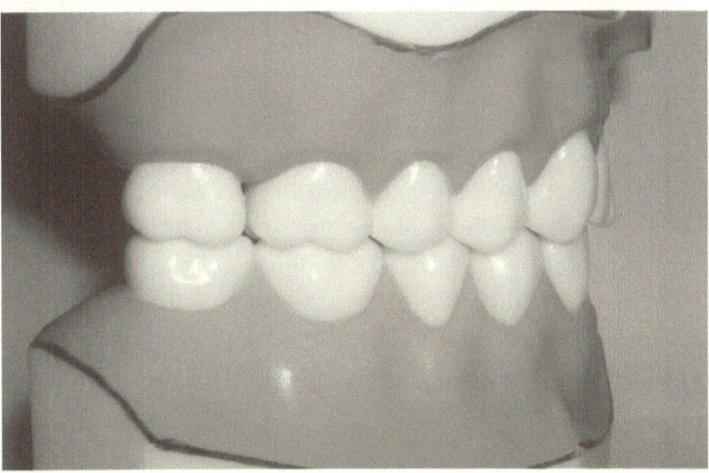

Fig. 10.1. Outside surfaces of posterior teeth and gums and upper and lower jaws Photo by Richard Coburn

If you open wide, your cheek muscles will be taut and you will only be able to get back as far as your first molar teeth. To get to the very back teeth, top and bottom and both sides close your mouth slightly, let the muscles of your cheeks and lips relax. Then you can get the bristles and paste to the very back teeth and gums easily.

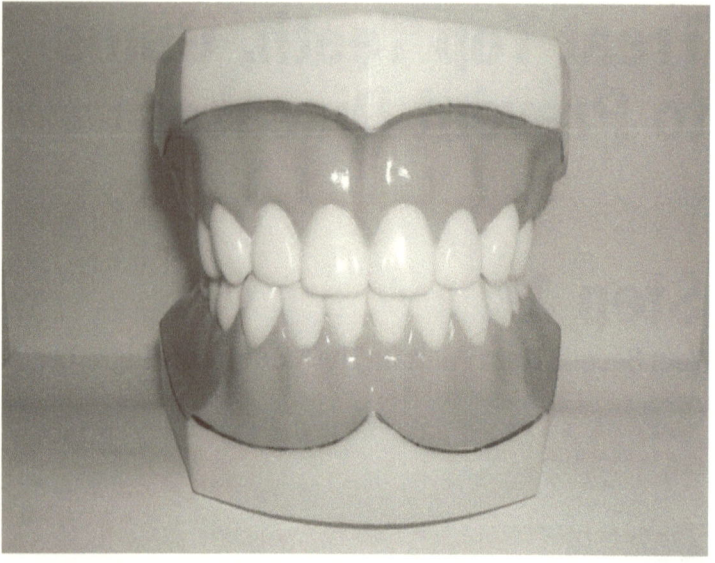

Fig. 10.2. Outside teeth and gum surfaces of front teeth
Photo by Richard Coburn

Hold the mouthtreater horizontally and move the bristles up and down vertically across the tooth surfaces and the gum surfaces up as far as the cheek or in the front up as far as the lip.

Continue all the way around from last molar tooth on one side across the front teeth and until you reach the last molar tooth on the other side.

Next, open wide, holding the mouthtreater horizontally with handle forward, pass the bristles backwards and forwards across the chewing surfaces of your back teeth, both sides. Then move the bristles from side to side across the back surface of the last tooth and gum behind it on each side.

Step 2

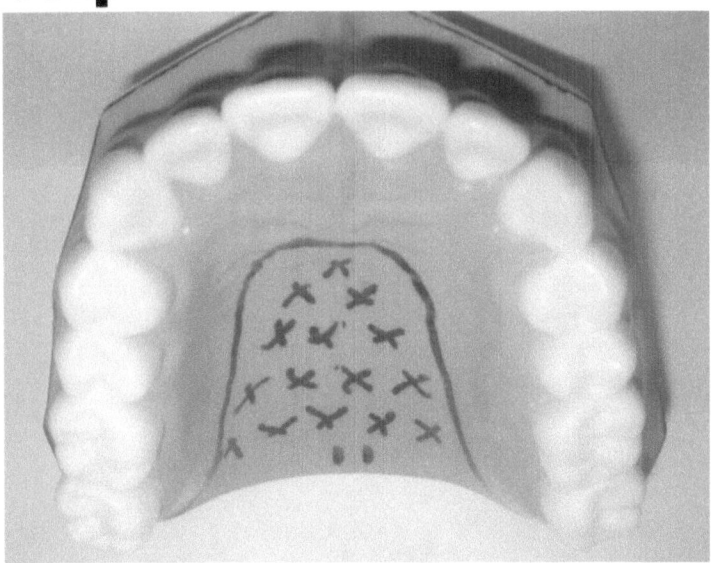

Fig. 10.3. Upper jaw: Chewing and inside surfaces of teeth and gums. Photo by Richard Coburn

Next, the inside surfaces of your top teeth and gums. Hold the mouthtreater vertically, handle down. Move the bristles across the surfaces of the teeth and across the gum to where the gum and the roof surfaces join. Continue all the way round from one side to the other.

CHAPTER **11**

Treat Bottom Teeth & Gums to Prevent Disease

Step 3

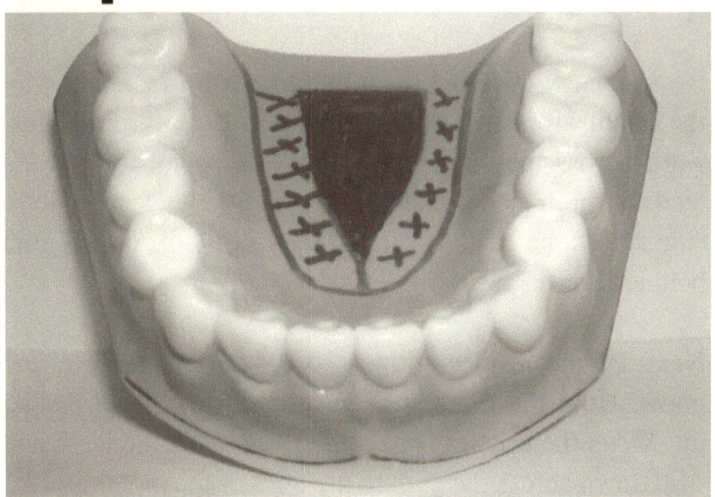

Fig. 11.1. Lower jaw: Outside and inside surfaces of teeth and gums and chewing surfaces of teeth. Photo by Richard Coburn

Next, you will treat the outside surfaces of your bottom teeth and gums. Remember to close your mouth a little to relax your cheek and lip muscles so the bristles can reach across the entire surfaces of the very back teeth and gum, all the way down to where the gum joins the cheeks and the lip.

Hold the mouthtreater horizontally with the handle forward. Move the bristles up and down vertically across the tooth surfaces and the gum surfaces, down as far as the cheek. Continue all the way around from the last molar tooth on one side, across the front teeth down to the lip, and to the last molar tooth on the other side.

Note particularly that you must relax your lip muscles to enable the bristles to reach down to the bottom of your gums; otherwise, as most people do, you will only succeed in the bristles touching the tips of your bottom front teeth.

Now, open wide. Hold the mouthtreater horizontally with the handle forward. Pass the bristles backward and forward across the chewing surfaces of your bottom back teeth on both sides. Then move the bristles from side to side across the back surface of the last tooth and the gum behind it on each side.

Next are the insides surfaces of your bottom teeth and gums. Hold the mouthtreater vertically with the handle up. Move the bristles across the surfaces of the teeth and well down across the gum to the floor of the mouth, all the way round from one side to the other.

CHAPTER **12**

Treat Tongue to Prevent Diseases

Step 4

Next, poke out your tongue and, starting at the tip, pass the bristles from side to side across the tongue. Repeat this for as far back on the tongue as you can tolerate. Then treat the tongue from front to back, again, as far back as you can tolerate.

Remember, after you have repeated this second treat, you will have painted the mouthpaste ingredients onto the already cleaned surfaces.

Look particularly at the mouth model pictures in the previous chapters to make absolutely certain you have cleaned and protected the very back surfaces of the last back teeth and gums, both upper and lower. You need to move the bristles from side to side for these surfaces to get the best results.

This entire process will have coated the surfaces of teeth, gums, and tongue with the beneficial ingredients in the mouthpaste. But let's take one more step to be sure.

CHAPTER **13**

Complete Second Treat to Prevent Disease

Step 5

After completing these next steps, *do not rinse with water!*

- Close your lips

- Thoroughly swish the foam repeatedly around and around inside your mouth

- Suck the foam repeatedly in and out between your teeth

- Spit out the excess foam

- Rinse the mouthtreater under the tap

That's it!

You have successfully treated your whole mouth: one treatment to clean every surface and a second to apply all the helpful ingredients in the mouthpaste to all surfaces inside of your mouth.

Your whole mouth will feel fresher than ever before. Your whole mouth will stay fresher for longer than ever before. Your entire oral cavity, every surface in it, is properly protected to prevent easily preventable oral diseases.

CHAPTER **14**

Counting The Costs of "The Rot"

Oral diseases are the most commonly occurring of all diseases. The ramifications of acute oral diseases and of chronic oral diseases, especially of tooth decay, acute gum disease, and chronic gum disease, are numerous and widely recorded. Here are just a very few general ramifications of "the Rot":

- Poor general health[1]

- Premature births

- Diabetes

- Loss of self-esteem[2]

- Lack of confidence

- Emotional problems[3]

- Poor employment prospects[4]

- Fear of dental treatment[5]

- Absenteeism from school and work[6]

- Massive social and economic costs born by governments[7]

- Prospects of having to choose between dental treatment services.[8] (Many people simply cannot afford the costs associated with some services and have to choose another service based on affordability, not preference, or have to defer treatment or never receive treatment.)

Perhaps the most serious ramifications of the Rot are the connections between oral diseases and the various forms of cardiovascular diseases.

A recent news item by Marlowe Hood, "Brush your teeth to avoid heart attacks," stated: "Heart disease is the No. 1 killer worldwide, claiming upward of 17 million lives every year, according to the World Health Organisation."[9, 10] The same article cites two independent researchers who recently confirmed the links between oral diseases and the various forms of cardiovascular diseases:

> *We now recognize that bacterial infections are an independent risk factor for heart diseases" said Professor Howard Jenkinson of the University of*

Bristol in Britain, at a meeting of the Society for General Microbiology in Dublin and a further comment by Steve Kerrigan of the Royal College of Surgeons in Dublin stated "The mouth is probably the dirtiest place in the human body.[11]

In separate research, a team led by Professor Greg Seymour of the University of Otago Dunedin in New Zealand showed how other bacteria in the mouth can provoke atherosclerosis, a disease that causes hardening of the arteries.[12]

(Author comment: Professor Jenkinson's press release ended with him making the following statement: "We are currently in the process of identifying the exact site at which the bacteria stick to the platelets. Once this is identified we will design a new drug to prevent this interaction." I wish the new drug every success for those who have need for it, but I wish even more that children will learn to prevent the offending oral diseases by treating their whole mouths as I advocate throughout this book.)

After reading the references above and as the author of "Stop the Rot," I absolutely and firmly believe that the instruction to Brush Your Teeth has been contributing to and will continue to contribute to oral diseases and to each of the ramifications stated above. If children are to be given a better chance to prevent oral diseases and their ramifications, they must be educated to Treat Your Whole Mouth.

Finally, there are considerable, and easily avoidable, dollar costs associated with the need for dental procedures and the treatment of oral diseases. Here is a sample of a few dental treatment services offered by dentists and an average estimated dollar amount charged for each service:

- Diagnostic services: comprehensive oral examination, $50; periodic oral examination, $42; oral exam limited, $39; intra-oral radiograph, $34

- Preventive services: removal of plaque or stain, $49; removal of calculus (scale), $49; external bleaching per tooth, $79; topical application of fluoride, $48; fissure sealing per tooth, $44; oral hygiene instruction, $31

- Oral surgery: removal of tooth, $126; surgical removal of tooth, $233

- Endodontics: root canal preparation, one canal, $202; root canal preparation, each additional canal, $93; root canal obturation, one canal, $196; root canal preparation, each additional canal, $92

- Restorative services: metallic restorations, depending on the number of surfaces, $100–$188; adhesive (white) restorations, depending on the number of surfaces, $109–$230; veneer facing, direct, $248; veneer facing, indirect, $804

- Prosthetics (dentures): full crown, $1194; bridge per pontic, $956; full crown fitted to osseointegrated implant, $1438; complete upper or lower\denture, $895;

> complete upper and lower dentures, $1595; partial plastic denture, $748; partial metal framed denture, $1138

Some people simply cannot afford the costs associated with some services and have to choose another service based on affordability, not preference. Some even have to defer treatment altogether.

Note the low cost associated with "oral hygiene instruction, $31." If the oral hygiene instruction happens to be Brush Your Teeth, that relic from the past, the advice is poor, out-of-date, and there should be no cost charged. Worst of all, by taking that advice, you will continue to be prone to ongoing oral diseases that will require ongoing treatment with the associated ongoing costs.

The dental profession has always offered the public the best and the most up-to-date dental services available for the treatment of oral diseases. They have been aided and well supported by fringe dental industries, the suppliers of dental materials and dental equipment. Together, they have made some important inroads into the prevention of oral diseases. In addition, fluoridation of water supplies, fluoride added to toothpastes, and fissure sealants placed in chewing surfaces of back teeth have all contributed to a dramatic reduction in the incidence of tooth decay.

But tooth decay is only one of the oral diseases children and adults should be able to prevent. What is being done about gum diseases and bad breath? Very little in my opinion. As for stained teeth, treating the problem has been met with great gusto by both the dental profession and dental manufacturers, but very little has been done about preventing it. Their oral health promotions and campaigns are good examples of their resistance to change advice to prevent oral diseases.[13, 14]

Just prior to self-publishing my first MouthWise Oral Health-Care Education resources in early 2002, I sent out information, such as you read in this book, on these resources to several dental associations around the world: the World Health Organization, numerous local dentists, politicians, education departments and to schools. The consistent reply was an emphatic silence. In several press releases since then my information has spread to several countries around the world. I have accused the dental profession of withholding important information from the public. In the last two or three years, two toothpaste and toothbrush manufacturers have marketed new products very closely based on my information. Why the silence from the others?

There is no doubt that there will be a negative financial impact on the entire dental industry if I can successfully convince parents, schools and teachers to stop telling children to brush your teeth and instead to accept my advice to instruct them to treat your whole mouth. That could be the reason for their silence.

Only you can decide between your two choices: Brush Your Teeth or Treat Your Whole Mouth. But when making that decision, please remember what Andy Warhol said:

"They always say time changes things, but you actually have to change them yourself."

Please, whomever you are, when giving children oral hygiene instructions, be certain those instructions, if followed, will prevent oral diseases and their ramifications with the greatest of certainty for the rest of those children's lives.

1. Mississippi Health Policy Research Center, "Children's Oral Health in Mississippi: Addressing a Silent Epidemic," *Centers for Disease Control and Prevention*, www.cdc.gov/oralhealth/publications/library/burden-book/pdfs/MS_policy_Brief.pdf.
2. www.oralhealthamerica.org/pdf/Disparitycavity.pdf.
3. See note 1.
4. See note 2.
5. Wikipedia, "Dental Fear," *Wikipedia*, http://en.wikipedia.org/wiki/Dento-phobia.
6. See note 2.
7. www.nidcr.nih.gov/DataStatistics/SurgeonGeneral/Report/Executive-Summary.htm.
8. www.ada.org.au/app_cmslib/media/lib/0702/m44810_v1_oral%20health%20expenditureOCT_06.pdf.
9. 12. Marlowe Hood, "Brush your teeth to avoid heart attacks," *News.com.au*, www.news.com.au/story/0,23599,24328823-23109,00.html.
10. www.who.int/cardiovascular_diseases/en.
11. www.bris.ac.uk/news/2008/5880.html.
12. http://dentistry.otago.ac.nz/news/media/mr0607_oralinfections.html.
13. Karen Fox, "ADA, Colgate team up for 'Save the World debut',https://www.ada.org/prof/resources/pubs/adanews/adanewsarticle.asprticleid=1058.
14. BDA, Colgate, "Healthy Teeth Require Healthy Gums", www.colgate.co.uk/app/OralHealthMonth/UK/Home.cvsp.

For additional reading on some of these topics, please refer to the following website pages:

- www.who.int/oral_health/media/en/orh_report03_en.pdf.
- www.cda-adc.ca/jcda/vol-67/issue-10/587.html.

CONCLUSION

In an early chapter, "Traditional Oral Hygiene Advice," I pointed out the flaws in the fifteenth-century, tooth-cleaning instruction to Brush Your Teeth, and I gave my reasons for why it can be a cause of oral diseases.

In another chapter, "Twenty-First Century MouthWise Oral Hygiene Advice," I stated that I had thought deeply about the following questions:

- What are the objectives of an ideal oral hygiene instruction?

- What oral hygiene instruction will best achieve these objectives?

- What is the best advice I can give to my patients to execute the instruction and achieve these objectives?

Subsequent chapters have detailed that I believe Treat Your Whole Mouth is the ideal oral hygiene instruction to give to children to prevent oral diseases.

I also believe the detailed advice I have given on how to Treat Your Whole Mouth is the very best advice children can receive to help them prevent easily preventable oral diseases with greater certainty than was ever possible with the instruction to Brush Your Teeth.

The greatest threats to children's oral health come from what children eat and drink. In this twenty-first century, sugar-laden, processed foods and drinks cause catastrophic damage in *every* mouth, but especially in children's mouths. When I began my work as a dentist, I used to see rot in teeth and gums every day. Fifty-five years later, I still see rot in teeth and gums every day.

Children have a habit of growing up to become adults. As adults, they continue to suffer from easily preventable oral diseases, especially from gum diseases that most people have regarded as acceptable and normal for adults. Not true! Most long-term, chronic gum disease results from the flawed instruction to Brush Your Teeth, which leaves the mouth dirty and unprotected. People do not realize that oral diseases result simply from mouths that were regarded as clean and protected from following Brush Your Teeth. Oral disease is preventable with simple, sensible, and total oral hygiene achieved only by treating your whole mouth.

Children grow up to have their own children, and they usually pass on the instructions they learned in childhood. Brush Your Teeth is one such instruction that has been passed on from generation to generation during every century for the past five centuries.

If, throughout this book, I have habitually repeated myself, I make no apologies. I simply hope it will remind you of the destruction and devastation created by the constant repetition of the tooth-cleaning instruction to Brush Your Teeth.

I sincerely hope I have convinced you to help me to ...

Stop the Rot! Stop Telling Children to "Brush Your Teeth"

Please note: The advice in this book is advice that, if taken, will positively impact a child's oral health for life, but it cannot be expected to reverse existing oral disease. If a child already has active oral diseases such as tooth decay or advanced gum disease, the child should be seen by a dentist as soon as possible for treatment. You must not expect all existing oral diseases to be resolved by adherence to Treat Your Mouth. However, giving children the ideal oral hygiene instruction to Treat Your Mouth may sometimes, and almost immediately, resolve minor gum diseases or even prevent the very early stages of tooth decay from advancing to the formation of cavities. Please make certain your child is orally fit when changing from Brush Your Teeth to Treat Your Mouth if your intention is to offer criticism at a later point in time.

Children deserve more than oral hygiene and healthcare instruction from their parents. They need an oral health education at school that is based on Treat Your Mouth. I firmly believe that children's teachers are their ideal oral health educators. I seek your help in achieving this for them. For details, please read the chapter titled "The Sensational Smiles Petition."

PUBLICATIONS

by the author

The 'MouthWise Oral HealthCare Manual 2'.

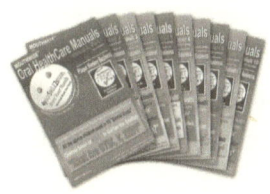

A printed set of 10 MouthWise Oral HealthCare Education Resources subtitled *'Visits 1 to 10 to GarGar The Dentist'*. For children aged 5 years to 11 years, for their parents and for their school teachers.

ISBN: 1-920712- 01- 1

The lesson for children in *Visit 1 to GarGar The Dentist* is titled "What Are STIX, Y, ZED?" Children learn about chemical elements, simple chemical compounds, and complex chemical compounds that they continually put into their mouths.

The lesson for children in *Visit 2 to GarGar The Dentist* is titled "Who Are STIX, Y, ZED?" Children are encouraged to look at food labels to identify ingredients in foods that they continually put into their mouths.

The lesson for children in *Visit 3 to GarGar The Dentist* is titled "Where Are STIX, Y, ZED in My Mouth?" Children learn about the basic anatomy of their teeth, gums, and tongue and where food and drinks can be found in their mouths after swallowing.

The lesson for children in *Visit 4 to GarGar The Dentist* is titled "X. Y. Z. PLAQUE and LURKEEZ." Children learn how plaque can form in their mouths and how the bacteria in the plaque can break down harmless chemical compounds into harmful, simple chemical elements.

The lesson for children in *Visit 5 to GarGar The Dentist* is titled "LURKEEZ and NASTEEZ." Children learn how plaque builds up in their mouths layer upon layer after each meal if it is not cleaned away and why this threatens their oral health.

The lesson for children in *Visit 6 to GarGar The Dentist* is titled "A Plaque Attack on Gums." Children learn how plaque can form scale on teeth and how gingivitis starts.

The lesson for children in *Visit 7 to GarGar The Dentist* is titled "A Plaque Attack on Teeth and Tongue." Children learn how tooth decay starts, how it can cause toothaches, and how it can eventually cause an abscess at the tip of the root.

The lesson for children in *Visit 8 to GarGar The Dentist* is titled "Harmful, Helpful and Harmless X. Y. Z." Children learn more about the chemicals they put into their mouths and are encouraged to avoid foods and drinks that are potentially harmful and to choose only foods and drinks that are either harmless or helpful.

The lesson for children in *Visit 9 to GarGar The Dentist* is titled "GarGar's ABC's of MouthWay Treat." In this lesson, children learn how to use mouthpaste and a mouth-treater to treat their mouths to prevent oral diseases.

The lesson for children in *Visit 10 to GarGar The Dentist* is titled "The MouthWay Treat Song Lyrics." Children learn the lyrics of the MouthWise Oral HealthCare oral hygiene song 4 Your Smile 2 Shine.

'4 Your Smile 2 Shine'

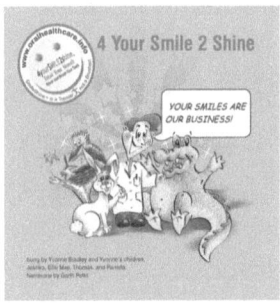

A MouthWise Oral HealthCare education resource that includes the narration of the ten lessons from *Visits 1 to 10 to GarGar The Dentist*, plus the lyrics and melody of the MouthWise Oral HealthCare Song *4 Your Smile 2 Shine*. The lyrics of the song are the MouthWise Oral Hygiene instruction for Treat Your Mouth. **ISBN: 1-920712- 12- 7**

The MouthWise Oral HealthCare Kit is the title given to a com- bined item that includes *MouthWise Oral HealthCare Manual*

2 and the CD *4 Your Smile 2 Shine.* A video available to MouthWise Members at www.mouthwisemouths.com gives this description of *The MouthWise Oral Health Kit:*

> *It's not easy teaching children the importance of good oral hygiene, and simply brushing your teeth has never eliminated oral diseases. Now you can make oral hygiene fun for kids with the MouthWise Oral Health Kit. This unique kit contains a set of ten books that best educates children on the basics of proper oral health care. Playful characters and fun-filled activities teach children ways to prevent oral diseases such as tooth decay, gum disease, and bad breath. Each book contains a quiz to test children's knowledge of what they have learned, plus a certificate of achievement for successfully completing each lesson. Also included is an informative CD, 4 Your Smile 2 Shine, that reinforces the message of good oral healthcare. Give your children a lifetime gift of whiter teeth, healthier gums, and fresher breath.*

The MouthWise Oral HealthCare School-on-the-Web is a downloadable teaching guideline resource for oral health-care educators. And anyone, even the untrained, can teach children the basics of good oral healthcare using *The MouthWise Oral HealthCare Kit.* Links to both can be found at www.oralhealthhelpsite.com.

Both the N.T. Education Curriculum Services and the Queensland Education Library Services have reviewed and recommended for use in primary schools the following MouthWise Oral HealthCare Education Resources:

- *The MouthWise Oral HealthCare School-on-the-Web* at www.oralhealthhelpsite.com

- *The MouthWise Oral HealthCare Manual 2*, ISBN: 1-920712-01-1

- The CD titled *4 Your Smile 2 Shine*, ISBN: 1-920712-12- 7

The MouthWise™ Oral Hygiene instruction "Treat Your Mouth" was published in 2002 in *The MouthWise Oral HealthCare Manual 2* for primary-aged children, their parents, and their teachers.

Sensational Smiles: Simple Advice 4 Your Smile 2 Shine from Teenage to Old Age, ISBN 978-1-60037-373-2. Published by Morgan James Publishing, New York, May 2008. Paperback.

WEBSITES

Current Websites of 4 Your Smile 2 Shine Pty Ltd.

www.mouthwiseshopping.com:
Online shopping for MouthWise Oral HealthCare Education Resources.

www.oralhealthhelpsite.com:
A MouthWise Oral HealthCare e-commerce and information site.

www.mouthwiselife.com:
A MouthWise Oral HealthCare site particularly for parents.

www.allaboutasmile.com:
A MouthWise Oral HealthCare site particularly for children.

www.Prevent-Oral-Disease-in-Children.blogspot.com:
My first blog site.

Websites Coming Soon in December 2008

The following websites will be incorporated into www. mouthwisemouths.com:

www.DrGarthPettit.com:
My personal blog site

www.MouthWiseMembers.com

www.StopTheRotStopTellingChildrenBrushYourTeeth.com

PETITION

The Sensational Smiles Petition

On May 1, 2008, my publisher, Morgan James Publishing, New York, released my book *Sensational Smiles: Simple Advice 4 Your Smile 2 Shine from Teenage to Old Age*, ISBN 978-1-60037-373-2.

In this book, I announced "The Sensational Smiles Petition," which reads as follows: "Oral health education based on 'Treat Your Whole Mouth,' not based on 'Brush Your Teeth,' should be mandatory for all children."

Please sign this petition.

You can get more information and sign "The Sensational Smiles Petition" at my website: www.MouthWiseLife.com.

Thank you very much,

Garth Pettit

Educating Children to "Treat Your Whole Mouth"

Parents, schools, and teachers have been innocent perpetrators of the oral diseases that routinely afflict children; diseases that often continue throughout their lives as I explain in my recent book, *Sensational Smiles: Simple Advice 4 Your Smile 2 Shine from Teen Age to Old Age*. I say "innocent perpetrators" because they have only been doing what they were told to do by the dental profession—telling children to "Brush Your Teeth."

Children are entitled to an oral health education, and it is imperative they receive one if they are to be given a chance to prevent oral diseases throughout their lifetimes.

The best oral health education that children can receive is education based on the oral hygiene instruction to "Treat Your Whole Mouth," not based on the old instruction to Brush Your Teeth.

Educating children to Treat Your Whole Mouth by using MouthWise Oral HealthCare education resources is made very simple and easy for would-be MouthWise oral health educators. Lots of help is available to you. There are no barriers to becoming a MouthWise oral health educator.

- Be the oral healthcare educators, parents or teachers or whoever.

- Be the oral healthcare educators trained or wishing to be trained in the art of teaching oral health.

- Be the oral healthcare educators knowledgeable in the subject materials.

- Oral healthcare educators choose lesson times from any time of twenty-four hours of each day.

- Oral healthcare educators choose lesson times from any of seven days of each week.

- Oral healthcare educators choose lesson times from any of fifty-two weeks of each year.

- Oral healthcare educators choose Internet-based, MouthWise Oral HealthCare, back-up resources such as *The MouthWise Oral HealthCare School-on-the-Web.*

- Oral healthcare educators only have to purchase *The MouthWise Oral Health Kit.*

Educating children to Treat Your Whole Mouth by using MouthWise Oral HealthCare Education Resources is not only great fun for children but also is extremely rewarding for their educators.

MEMBERS

If you have been telling children, either as an individual or as part of an organization, to Brush Your Teeth and you wish to change to telling children to Treat Your Mouth or Treat Your Whole Mouth., please be advised there is help available when you become a MouthWise member. Becoming a member gives you access to some MouthWise Oral HealthCare education resources not available anywhere else. MouthWise Oral HealthCare education resources are continually in the process of being updated are added to.

People who would benefit most by becoming a Mouth-Wise Member would include:

- Parents
- Schools
- Classroom teachers
- Dental and allied professionals
- Individuals

The intended five levels of MouthWise Memberships are

- Free
- Bronze (USD$1 for lifetime)
- Silver (USD$10 per month)
- Gold (USD$15 per month)
- Platinum (USD$20 per month)

Not all levels are available at the time this book is going to print but will become available as soon as is possible.

Membership levels may be changed or cancelled at any time.

For all details of MouthWise Memberships please visit www.mouthwisemembers.com.

CREDITS

I dedicate this book, *Stop the Rot! Stop Telling Children to "Brush Your Teeth,"* to my deceased parents, Selina Trixie Pettit and George William Pettit, who gave me an idyllic childhood filled with love and happiness and who always encouraged the achievement of any goal so long as it was morally correct. In the past twelve years, while creating the MouthWise Oral HealthCare Education Resources, that philosophy has continuously strengthened my resolve to finish that which I set out to do—prevent oral disease in children!

MouthWise, MouthTreater, MouthPaste, Treat Your Mouth, Treat Your Whole Mouth, and 4 Your Smile 2 Shine. Are trademarks of Garth D Pettit, licensed to MouthWise Oral HealthCare, A division of 4 Your Smile 2 Shine Pty Ltd ABN 12 089 094 182

Published by: Morgan James Publishing, New York, USA

Illustrations by: Leonie Molloy of RedEye Media, Megan Spiers of mega-ART, C.D.A.A. of Adelaide, Richard Coburn at Acoustics in Art Media Productions

Author, Dr Garth Pettit BDS GDM

Distributed by Ingram Publishing Services

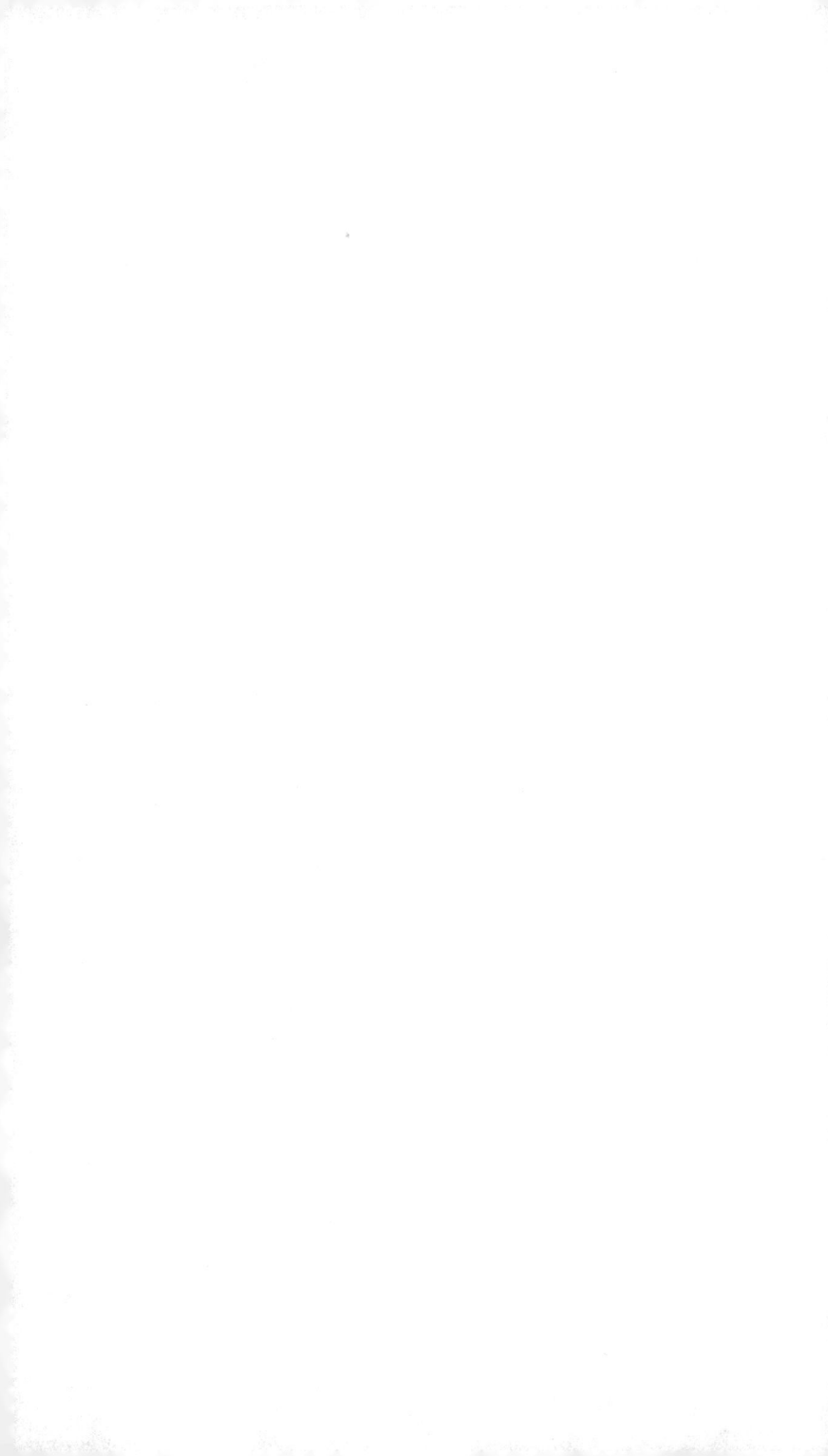